This publication is intended to provide educational information for the reader on the covered subjects. It is not intended to take the place of personalized medical counseling, diagnosis, and treatment from a trained healthcare professional.

ISBN 978-1-998740-17-8 (Paperback)
ISBN 978-1-998740-18-5 (eBook)

Printed and bound in USA
Published by Loons Press

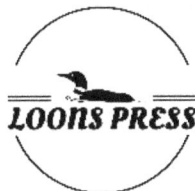

LOONS PRESS

Table Of Contents

How To Ease Restless Legs Syndrome

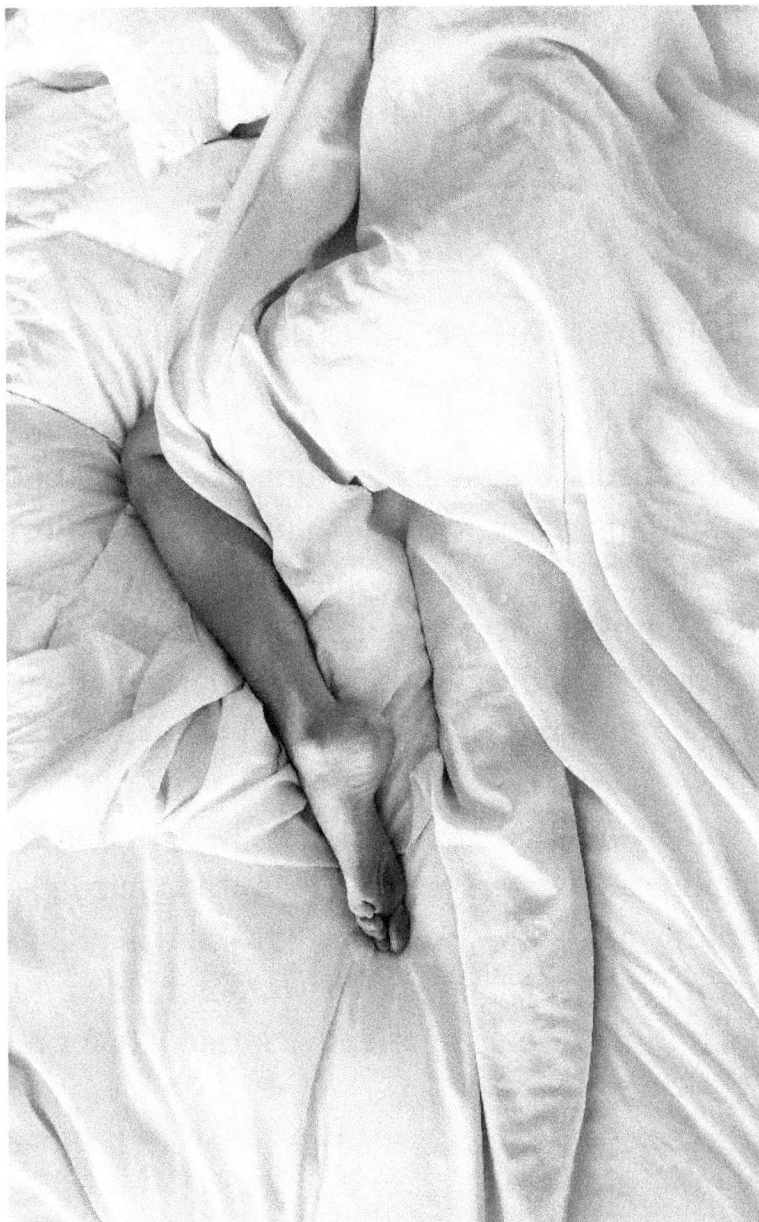

Effective Strategies for Relief

Chapter 1

Understanding Restless Legs Syndrome

Definition and Symptoms

Restless Legs Syndrome (RLS) is a neurological disorder characterized by an uncontrollable urge to move the legs, often accompanied by uncomfortable sensations. These sensations can include tingling, itching, burning, or crawling feelings that typically occur when an individual is at rest, particularly in the evening or at night.

This condition is not merely a habit or a psychological issue; rather, it is recognized as a legitimate medical disorder that can significantly impact a person's quality of life. Understanding RLS is crucial for those seeking effective strategies for relief.

The symptoms of RLS can vary widely among individuals, but the most common experience is a compelling urge to move the legs, which is often relieved temporarily by movement. This may involve pacing, stretching, or walking around, and the relief is usually short-lived, prompting individuals to feel the need to move again. In addition to the urge to move, many people with RLS report uncomfortable sensations in their legs that can disrupt sleep and lead to fatigue during the day. These sensations often worsen during periods of inactivity, making it difficult to sit for extended periods, such as during long car rides or while watching television.

Another significant aspect of RLS symptoms is their nocturnal nature. Many individuals find that their symptoms intensify in the evening, making it challenging to fall asleep or stay asleep. This can lead to a vicious cycle of insomnia, as the inability to rest properly exacerbates the symptoms. Sleep disturbances resulting from RLS not only impact physical well-being but can also contribute to emotional and mental fatigue, affecting overall quality of life. Recognizing this connection between RLS and sleep disruption is essential for understanding the broader implications of the disorder.

RLS is also associated with a range of secondary symptoms that may further complicate the condition. These can include anxiety and depression, which are often linked to the frustration and sleep deprivation caused by the syndrome. Some individuals may experience periodic limb movements during sleep (PLMS), which are involuntary jerking or twitching motions that occur during sleep and can further disrupt rest. Acknowledging these interconnected symptoms can help individuals and healthcare providers develop a comprehensive approach to managing RLS.

For those concerned about how to ease Restless Legs Syndrome, recognizing the definition and symptoms is the first step toward seeking effective relief strategies. With a clearer understanding of what RLS entails, individuals can better identify their symptoms and communicate effectively with healthcare professionals. This lays the groundwork for exploring various management techniques, including lifestyle changes, medical treatments, and alternative therapies, all aimed at alleviating the discomfort associated with this challenging condition.

Causes and Triggers

Restless Legs Syndrome (RLS) is a complex neurological disorder characterized by an uncontrollable urge to move the legs, often accompanied by uncomfortable sensations. Understanding the causes and triggers of RLS is crucial for those seeking effective strategies for relief. While the exact cause of RLS remains unclear, several factors have been identified that contribute to the onset and exacerbation of symptoms. Genetic predisposition plays a significant role, as RLS often runs in families, suggesting a hereditary component that can influence an individual's susceptibility to the condition.

Another significant factor in the development of RLS is the presence of underlying medical conditions. Disorders such as iron deficiency anemia, diabetes, and peripheral neuropathy have been linked to RLS. Iron deficiency, in particular, is noteworthy because iron is essential for dopamine production, which is a neurotransmitter involved in regulating movement. When iron levels are low, it can lead to disruptions in the brain's ability to control leg movements, worsening RLS symptoms.

Therefore, individuals with these medical conditions should work closely with their healthcare providers to address any deficiencies or complications that may aggravate their RLS.

Lifestyle choices also play a critical role in triggering and exacerbating RLS symptoms. Caffeine, nicotine, and alcohol are known to stimulate the nervous system, potentially worsening symptoms for individuals already prone to RLS. Additionally, sedentary behavior can contribute to the severity of symptoms.

Prolonged periods of inactivity may lead to increased discomfort, making it vital for those with RLS to incorporate regular movement and stretching into their daily routines. Identifying and modifying these lifestyle factors can be an effective strategy for managing symptoms.

Sleep disturbances are another common trigger for RLS. Many individuals with RLS experience difficulty falling asleep or staying asleep due to their symptoms, which can create a vicious cycle of fatigue and increased RLS severity.

Sleep deprivation can heighten the perception of discomfort in the legs, making it essential for individuals with RLS to prioritize good sleep hygiene. Establishing a regular sleep schedule, creating a comfortable sleep environment, and avoiding stimulants before bedtime can help mitigate sleep-related triggers.

Finally, hormonal changes, particularly in women, can influence the severity of RLS symptoms. Many women report that their symptoms worsen during pregnancy or during hormonal fluctuations associated with their menstrual cycle. These hormonal influences may alter neurotransmitter levels and increase sensitivity in the legs.

Understanding these triggers can empower individuals to anticipate flare-ups and take proactive measures to manage their symptoms effectively. By recognizing the myriad causes and triggers of RLS, individuals can better equip themselves to seek appropriate treatment and adopt lifestyle changes that promote relief.

The Impact on Daily Life

Restless Legs Syndrome (RLS) significantly impacts daily life for those affected by it, creating challenges that extend beyond mere discomfort. Individuals with RLS often experience an uncontrollable urge to move their legs, particularly during periods of inactivity or at night. This compulsion can lead to sleep disturbances, decreased productivity, and heightened stress levels. The condition not only disrupts the individual's comfort but also affects relationships, as family members and friends may struggle to understand the symptoms and their implications.

Sleep is one of the most affected aspects of daily life for those with RLS. The urge to move the legs can make it difficult to fall asleep or maintain restful sleep, leading to chronic fatigue. This fatigue often manifests as irritability, difficulty concentrating, and diminished cognitive function. As a result, individuals may find it challenging to perform at their best in professional or academic settings. The struggle for restorative sleep can create a cycle of exhaustion that exacerbates the symptoms of RLS, making it essential to address both the syndrome and its sleep-related consequences.

In addition to sleep disturbances, RLS can impact social interactions and leisure activities. Individuals may avoid situations that require prolonged sitting, such as watching movies, attending concerts, or even traveling. This avoidance can lead to social isolation, as the fear of experiencing symptoms in public may deter individuals from participating in enjoyable activities. The resultant isolation can foster feelings of loneliness and depression, compounding the psychological burden of living with RLS.

Moreover, managing RLS often requires lifestyle adjustments that can further alter daily routines. Individuals may need to implement strategies such as regular exercise, dietary changes, and stress management techniques.

While these strategies can provide relief, the effort required to maintain them can feel overwhelming at times. The necessity for constant vigilance regarding triggers can also lead to anxiety, as individuals worry about when and where symptoms may arise, affecting their ability to enjoy spontaneous moments in life.

Understanding the impact of RLS on daily life is crucial for developing effective management strategies. Individuals experiencing RLS must recognize that they are not alone in their struggles and that there are numerous approaches to alleviate symptoms.

By addressing the condition holistically—considering its effects on sleep, social life, and daily routines—those affected can take proactive steps toward improving their quality of life. Empowering oneself with knowledge and support can help mitigate the challenges posed by RLS and foster a more fulfilling existence.

How To Ease Restless Legs Syndrome

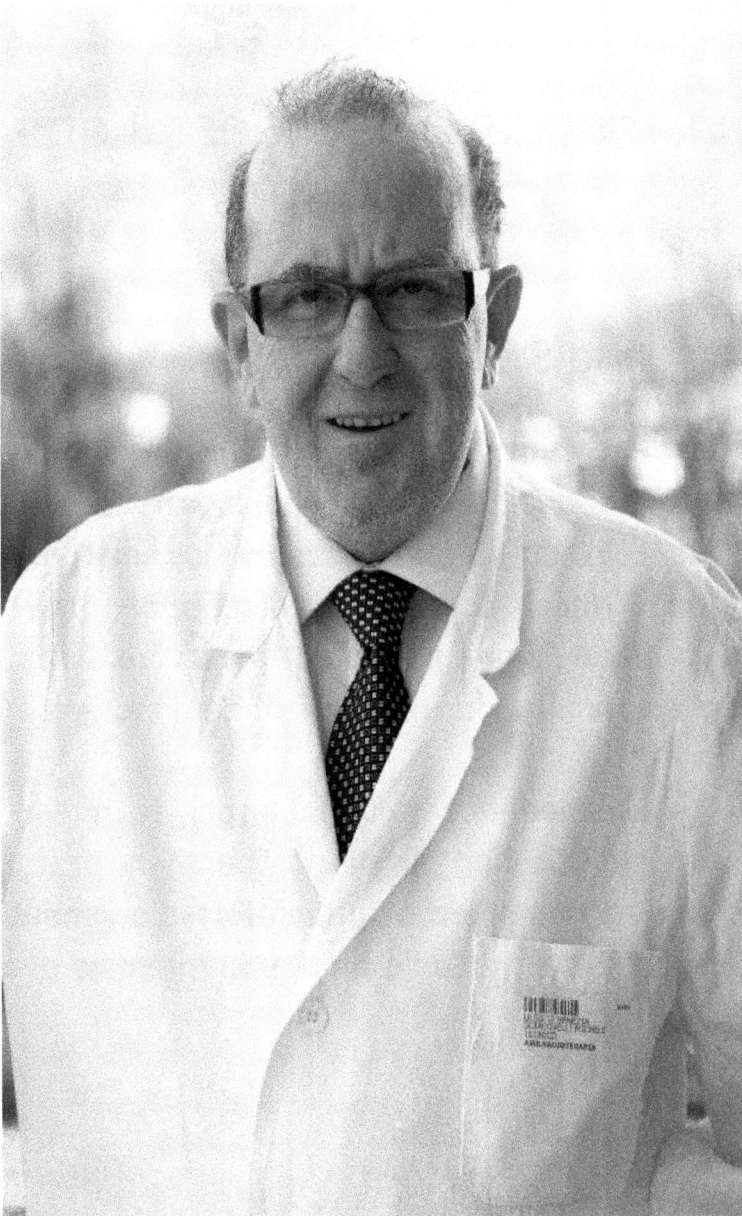

Effective Strategies for Relief

Chapter 2

Diagnosis of Restless Legs Syndrome

When to See a Doctor

Restless Legs Syndrome (RLS) can significantly impact one's quality of life, making it essential to understand when it is necessary to seek medical attention. While occasional discomfort may be manageable at home, persistent or severe symptoms warrant a consultation with a healthcare professional.

If you experience frequent urges to move your legs, especially during periods of inactivity, or if these urges are accompanied by uncomfortable sensations, it is advisable to schedule an appointment to discuss your symptoms.

Another critical indicator for seeing a doctor is the frequency and duration of your symptoms. If you find that your restless legs are interrupting your sleep or daily activities multiple times a week, this may indicate a more serious underlying issue that needs addressing.

Chronic sleep disturbances can lead to fatigue, mood changes, and difficulty concentrating, further exacerbating the impact of RLS on your life. A healthcare provider can help assess the severity of your condition and determine the best course of action.

Consider seeking medical advice if you notice that your symptoms are progressively worsening. If the discomfort in your legs becomes more intense or starts to occur during the day, it may signal that RLS is evolving and could require more targeted treatment. Additionally, if you have tried over-the-counter remedies or lifestyle changes without any improvement, a doctor can offer alternative solutions or medications that may be more effective for your specific situation.

For individuals with a history of other medical conditions, such as diabetes, kidney disease, or neuropathy, it is crucial to consult a healthcare provider sooner rather than later. RLS can sometimes be a symptom of an underlying health issue, and addressing these conditions may alleviate your restless legs.

A comprehensive evaluation can help identify any contributing factors and tailor a management plan that considers all aspects of your health.

Lastly, if you experience any unusual symptoms in conjunction with RLS, such as swelling, pain, or skin changes in your legs, it is imperative to see a doctor promptly. These symptoms could indicate complications that require immediate attention.

Being proactive about your health and seeking medical advice when necessary can lead to better management of RLS and improve overall well-being.

Diagnostic Criteria

Restless Legs Syndrome (RLS) is a neurological disorder characterized by an uncontrollable urge to move the legs, often accompanied by uncomfortable sensations. Understanding the diagnostic criteria for RLS is essential for individuals who suspect they may be affected by this condition. The criteria established by the International Restless Legs Syndrome Study Group serve as a guideline for healthcare providers in accurately diagnosing RLS. These criteria help distinguish RLS from other conditions that may mimic its symptoms, allowing for appropriate management and relief strategies.

The first key criterion for diagnosing RLS is the presence of an overwhelming urge to move the legs. This sensation is typically described as uncomfortable, with patients often reporting feelings of crawling, tingling, or aching. Importantly, this urge tends to worsen during periods of inactivity, such as sitting or lying down, prompting individuals to seek relief through movement. The urge must also be associated with discomfort that can be temporarily relieved by movement, highlighting the unique nature of RLS compared to other leg-related conditions.

Another critical aspect of the diagnostic criteria involves the timing of symptoms. For a diagnosis of RLS to be confirmed, symptoms must occur primarily in the evening or at night, which often leads to significant sleep disturbances. Patients may find themselves unable to relax or fall asleep due to the uncomfortable sensations, resulting in daytime fatigue and impaired quality of life. Evaluating the timing and frequency of these symptoms is crucial in establishing a correct diagnosis and ensuring that appropriate treatment options are considered.

Additionally, the diagnostic criteria stipulate that the symptoms must not be better explained by other medical or behavioral conditions. Various disorders, including peripheral neuropathy, arthritis, and sleep apnea, can present with similar symptoms. Therefore, healthcare providers will often conduct a thorough medical history and physical examination, alongside relevant tests, to rule out alternative causes. This comprehensive approach ensures that patients receive an accurate diagnosis and tailored treatment plan that addresses their specific needs.

Finally, it is essential to recognize that the severity of RLS symptoms can vary widely among individuals. Some may experience mild discomfort that is manageable, while others may suffer from severe symptoms that significantly disrupt daily activities and sleep. Evaluating the impact of RLS on a person's life is vital in determining the most effective strategies for relief. By understanding the diagnostic criteria for RLS, individuals can better communicate their symptoms to healthcare providers, paving the way for an accurate diagnosis and an effective management plan tailored to their unique situation.

Common Misdiagnoses

Restless Legs Syndrome (RLS) is often misdiagnosed as other conditions, leading to prolonged discomfort and ineffective treatments. One of the most common misdiagnoses is that of peripheral neuropathy. Patients experiencing the uncomfortable sensations associated with RLS may be mistakenly identified as having nerve damage, which can result from diabetes or other underlying health issues.

This misinterpretation can lead to inappropriate treatments focusing on nerve regeneration rather than addressing the root cause of the restless legs.

Another frequent misdiagnosis occurs with anxiety disorders. Many individuals with RLS report feelings of anxiety or restlessness, which can lead healthcare providers to attribute their symptoms to anxiety rather than a neurological condition. This misclassification can cause patients to undergo unnecessary psychological evaluations and treatments. It's crucial to recognize that while anxiety may coexist with RLS, it is not the primary cause of the leg discomfort that characterizes this syndrome.

RLS is also sometimes confused with general insomnia or sleep disorders. While it is true that the symptoms of RLS often worsen during periods of inactivity, leading to difficulties in falling or staying asleep, the underlying issue is distinct. Insomnia treatments may alleviate some of the sleep disruption but will not address the uncomfortable sensations in the legs that trigger the need to move. Patients who find themselves caught in this cycle may continue to suffer without receiving the appropriate diagnosis and treatment for RLS.

Another condition that can be misdiagnosed alongside RLS is arthritis or joint pain. Individuals may attribute their leg discomfort to arthritis, especially if they have a history of joint issues. However, RLS symptoms are characterized by specific sensations that are not typically associated with joint pain. Treatments aimed at managing arthritis will likely not provide relief for the sensory symptoms of RLS, further complicating the patient's experience and prolonging their suffering.

Recognizing the potential for misdiagnosis is vital for effective management of Restless Legs Syndrome. Awareness of these common pitfalls can empower patients to advocate for themselves and seek further evaluation when initial diagnoses do not lead to improvement. By understanding the distinct nature of RLS and its symptoms, individuals can ensure they receive targeted treatment strategies, leading to more effective relief from their discomfort.

How To Ease Restless Legs Syndrome

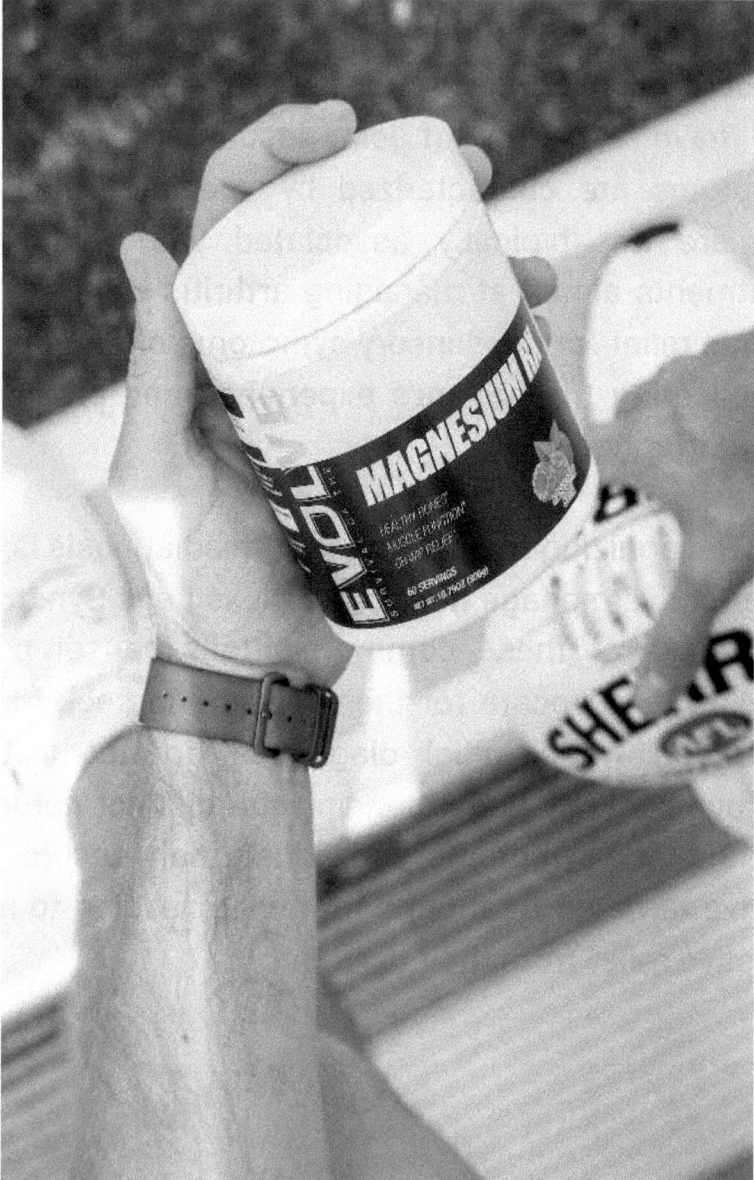

Chapter 3

Lifestyle Changes for Relief

Diet and Nutrition

Diet and nutrition play a crucial role in managing Restless Legs Syndrome (RLS). While the exact causes of RLS are not fully understood, certain dietary choices can significantly impact the severity of symptoms. A well-balanced diet rich in essential nutrients can help alleviate some discomfort associated with RLS.

Key nutrients to focus on include iron, magnesium, and folate, which are vital for proper nerve function and overall health. Incorporating foods high in these nutrients may contribute to reduced symptoms and improved quality of life.

Iron is particularly important for individuals with RLS, as low iron levels are often linked to the condition. Foods such as lean meats, fish, poultry, legumes, and dark leafy greens should be included in the diet to boost iron intake.

For those who may struggle to absorb iron from plant sources, pairing them with vitamin C-rich foods can enhance absorption. It is advisable to monitor iron levels through blood tests and consult with a healthcare professional before making significant dietary changes or starting supplements.

Magnesium is another essential mineral that can help ease RLS symptoms. This nutrient plays a role in muscle function and relaxation, making it beneficial for those experiencing leg discomfort. Foods such as nuts, seeds, whole grains, and bananas are excellent sources of magnesium. Maintaining adequate magnesium levels may help reduce muscle cramps and promote a sense of calm, which can be particularly helpful during the evening hours when RLS symptoms often worsen.

Folate, a B vitamin, is also linked to nerve health and can aid individuals with RLS. Incorporating foods high in folate, such as fortified cereals, beans, and citrus fruits, can help maintain adequate levels. Additionally, staying well-hydrated is crucial, as dehydration can exacerbate RLS symptoms.

It is essential to drink enough water throughout the day while being mindful of caffeine and alcohol intake, as these can disrupt sleep and worsen symptoms.

Overall, adopting a balanced diet that prioritizes essential nutrients like iron, magnesium, and folate can be a significant step towards managing Restless Legs Syndrome. Individuals should consider keeping a food diary to track their dietary habits and identify potential triggers for their symptoms. By focusing on nutrition and making informed dietary choices, individuals can take proactive steps toward easing their RLS symptoms and enhancing their overall well-being.

Exercise and Physical Activity

Exercise and physical activity play a crucial role in managing Restless Legs Syndrome (RLS). Engaging in regular physical activity can alleviate symptoms and improve overall well-being. Activities such as walking, cycling, and swimming can enhance circulation and reduce the sensations associated with RLS.

It is important to find an exercise routine that suits individual preferences and capabilities. Consistency is key, as regular movement can help mitigate the discomfort that often accompanies this condition.

Low-impact exercises are particularly beneficial for individuals with RLS. These activities minimize strain on the body while promoting blood flow and muscle relaxation. Gentle stretching exercises can also be effective, as they help to loosen tight muscles and reduce tension in the legs. Incorporating flexibility and balance training, such as yoga or tai chi, can further enhance physical health and provide mental relaxation. These practices have been shown to reduce stress, which is a known trigger for RLS symptoms.

Timing of exercise is another important factor to consider. While regular physical activity is beneficial, exercising too close to bedtime may exacerbate symptoms for some individuals. It is advisable to schedule workouts earlier in the day to allow the body ample time to wind down before sleep. Finding the right balance and listening to one's body can help optimize the benefits of exercise without aggravating RLS symptoms.

In addition to structured exercise, increasing overall daily movement can contribute to relief from RLS symptoms. Simple changes, such as taking short walks during breaks, using stairs instead of elevators, or engaging in household chores, can enhance physical activity levels.

These small adjustments can have a cumulative effect, leading to improved circulation and reduced discomfort in the legs.

Lastly, it is important to consult with healthcare professionals before starting any new exercise program, especially for those with pre-existing health conditions. A tailored exercise plan that considers individual health status and preferences can be developed with professional guidance.

By incorporating regular physical activity into their lifestyle, individuals with Restless Legs Syndrome can experience significant improvements in their symptoms and overall quality of life.

Sleep Hygiene

Sleep hygiene refers to a series of practices and habits that are conducive to sleeping well on a regular basis. For individuals dealing with Restless Legs Syndrome (RLS), maintaining good sleep hygiene can significantly enhance the quality of sleep and reduce the severity of symptoms. Establishing a consistent sleep routine is one of the foundational aspects of sleep hygiene.

This involves going to bed and waking up at the same time each day, even on weekends. A regular schedule helps regulate the body's internal clock, which can promote more restful sleep and reduce the frequency of RLS symptoms during the night.

Creating a comfortable sleep environment is another critical component of sleep hygiene. The bedroom should be conducive to sleep, which means keeping it dark, quiet, and cool. Consider using blackout curtains to block out light, white noise machines or earplugs to minimize disruptive sounds, and maintaining a comfortable temperature.

Additionally, investing in a comfortable mattress and pillows can greatly affect sleep quality. For those with RLS, the right sleeping position may also play a role in alleviating discomfort; finding a position that minimizes leg restlessness can be beneficial.

Limiting exposure to stimulants is essential for promoting better sleep hygiene, especially for individuals with RLS. Caffeine, nicotine, and certain medications can interfere with the ability to fall asleep and stay asleep. It is advisable to avoid these substances, particularly in the hours leading up to bedtime. Alcohol, while sometimes believed to aid sleep, can lead to disrupted sleep patterns and worsen RLS symptoms. Therefore, it is important to manage the intake of these substances to improve overall sleep quality.

Incorporating relaxation techniques before bedtime can also aid in improving sleep hygiene. Activities such as reading, gentle stretching, meditation, or taking a warm bath can help signal to the body that it is time to wind down. These practices can help reduce stress and anxiety, which are known to exacerbate RLS symptoms.

Establishing a calming pre-sleep routine can help prepare the mind and body for sleep, making it easier to drift off and remain asleep throughout the night.

Lastly, monitoring daytime activities can further enhance sleep hygiene and help manage RLS symptoms. Regular physical activity is beneficial, but it is essential to time workouts properly; exercising too close to bedtime can energize the body and make it difficult to fall asleep. Instead, aim for regular, moderate exercise earlier in the day.

Additionally, paying attention to dietary habits—such as maintaining a balanced diet and staying hydrated—can contribute to better sleep. By adopting these sleep hygiene practices, individuals with Restless Legs Syndrome can create a more favorable environment for sleep and potentially reduce the frequency and intensity of their symptoms.

How To Ease Restless Legs Syndrome

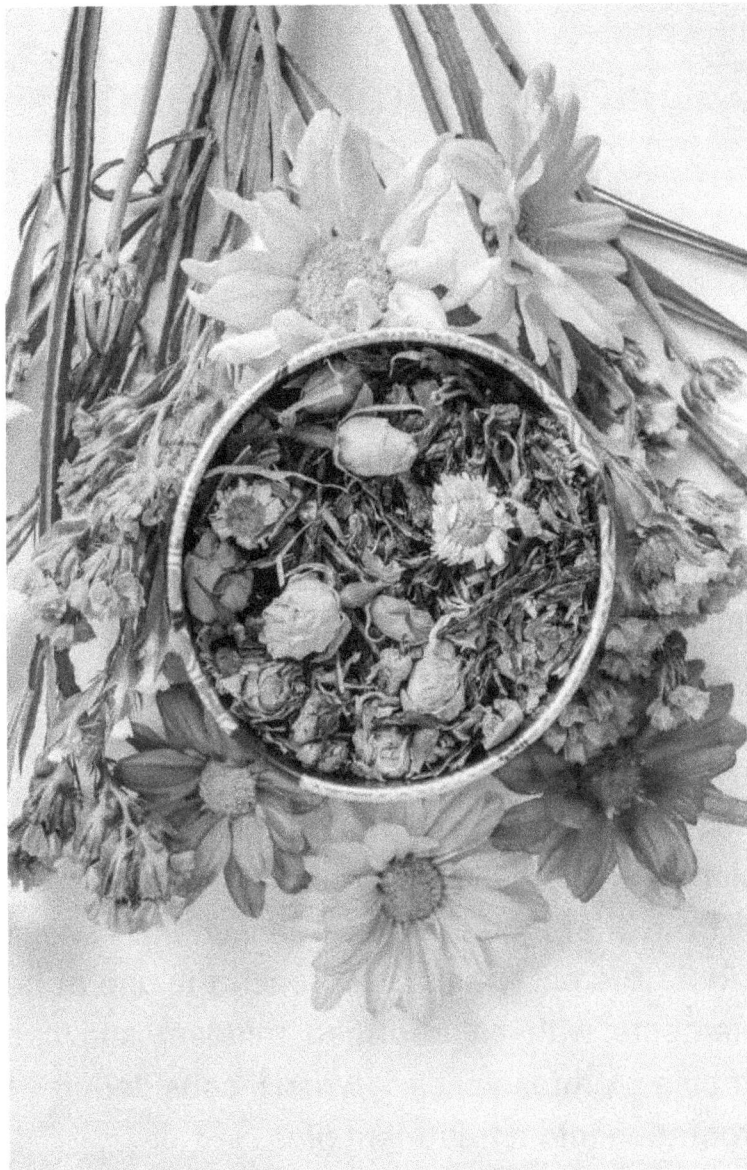

Chapter 4

Home Remedies and Natural Treatments

Herbal Supplements

Herbal supplements have gained popularity as potential remedies for various health conditions, including Restless Legs Syndrome (RLS). Many individuals suffering from RLS seek natural alternatives to pharmaceutical treatments, often turning to herbal remedies that have been used for centuries in traditional medicine.

While scientific research on the efficacy of these supplements is still evolving, some herbs may offer relief from the uncomfortable sensations associated with RLS. It is essential to approach the use of herbal supplements with an informed mindset and consult healthcare professionals when considering their incorporation into a treatment plan.

How To Ease Restless Legs Syndrome

One of the most commonly discussed herbal supplements for RLS is valerian root. Valerian is known for its sedative properties and has been used to promote relaxation and improve sleep quality. For individuals experiencing RLS symptoms primarily at night, valerian root may help alleviate the sensation of restless legs and enhance overall sleep. While some studies suggest that valerian can improve sleep quality, its direct effect on RLS symptoms requires further investigation. It is advisable to discuss valerian supplementation with a healthcare provider, especially for those already taking other medications.

Another herbal option is passionflower, which is often used to manage anxiety and improve sleep. This herb acts as a mild sedative and may help reduce the stress and anxiety that can exacerbate RLS symptoms. Some users report that passionflower helps them feel calmer and more relaxed, potentially minimizing the urge to move their legs. As with valerian, clinical evidence supporting the specific effectiveness of passionflower for RLS is limited, highlighting the importance of personal experimentation under professional guidance.

Ginger and turmeric are two other herbs that may benefit individuals with RLS, primarily due to their anti-inflammatory properties. Chronic inflammation can contribute to various health issues, including discomfort associated with RLS. Incorporating ginger or turmeric into the diet may help reduce inflammation, potentially alleviating some of the symptoms experienced by RLS sufferers. Both herbs can be consumed in various forms, including teas, capsules, or as part of cooked dishes.

However, those considering high doses or concentrated supplements should consult a healthcare provider to avoid adverse effects or interactions with other medications.

Finally, it is crucial for individuals to approach the use of herbal supplements with caution and realistic expectations. While some may find relief from RLS symptoms through herbal remedies, these supplements are not guaranteed solutions and may not work for everyone. A comprehensive treatment plan that includes lifestyle changes, dietary adjustments, and other therapies should be considered for managing RLS effectively.

Engaging with healthcare professionals knowledgeable about both conventional and alternative treatments can help individuals navigate their options and find the most suitable approach for their specific needs.

Essential Oils

Essential oils have gained popularity as a natural remedy for various health issues, including Restless Legs Syndrome (RLS). These concentrated extracts from plants possess unique therapeutic properties that may provide relief from the uncomfortable sensations associated with RLS. The use of essential oils can complement other treatment methods, offering a holistic approach to managing symptoms. By understanding the specific oils that can help and how to use them effectively, individuals can create a supportive environment for alleviating their discomfort.

One of the most commonly recommended essential oils for RLS is lavender. Known for its calming and relaxing properties, lavender essential oil can help ease tension and promote better sleep, which is often disrupted in individuals with RLS.

Applying diluted lavender oil to the legs or using it in a diffuser before bedtime may help to create a soothing atmosphere conducive to relaxation. Additionally, studies suggest that the aroma of lavender can reduce anxiety, further contributing to a sense of calm that may alleviate RLS symptoms.

Another essential oil that can be beneficial is peppermint. This oil is well-known for its invigorating scent and cooling effect, which can help relieve inflammation and soothe muscle discomfort. Massaging diluted peppermint oil into the legs may provide immediate relief from the restless sensations felt during the night. Furthermore, the stimulating properties of peppermint can enhance blood circulation, which is particularly beneficial for those experiencing poor circulation related to RLS.

Cypress essential oil is also noteworthy for its potential to alleviate symptoms of RLS. Its properties include promoting circulation and reducing muscle spasms, making it a valuable addition to an RLS management plan. When used in a massage blend, cypress oil can help to relieve the heaviness and discomfort often experienced in the legs.

Combining cypress with other oils, such as lavender or chamomile, can enhance its effectiveness, creating a synergistic effect that may result in greater relief.

Incorporating essential oils into a daily routine for managing RLS can be achieved through various methods. Aromatherapy diffusers, topical applications, and even baths with essential oils can provide opportunities for individuals to experience the benefits of these natural substances. It is essential to use high-quality, pure essential oils and to perform a patch test before applying them to the skin. Additionally, consulting with a healthcare professional before incorporating essential oils into an RLS treatment plan is prudent, ensuring that they align with individual health needs and conditions.

Warm and Cold Therapy

Warm and cold therapy are two complementary approaches that can provide significant relief for individuals suffering from Restless Legs Syndrome (RLS). Each method stimulates different bodily responses, which can help alleviate the uncomfortable sensations associated with RLS.

Understanding how to effectively use both therapies can empower individuals to manage their symptoms more effectively and enhance their overall quality of life.

Warm therapy typically involves the application of heat to soothe muscle tension and improve blood circulation. For those with RLS, applying warmth to the legs can help to ease the discomfort and reduce the urge to move. Common methods of warm therapy include warm baths, heating pads, and warm compresses. Taking a warm bath before bedtime can be particularly beneficial, as it not only relaxes the muscles but also prepares the body for sleep. The gentle heat promotes relaxation and can create a calming effect, making it easier to fall asleep without the nagging sensations that often accompany RLS.

On the other hand, cold therapy can also play a crucial role in managing RLS symptoms. Cold applications can numb the affected areas and reduce inflammation, providing a contrasting effect to heat therapy. Ice packs or cold compresses can be applied to the legs for short periods, helping to alleviate the discomfort that triggers the urge to move.

While cold therapy may not be as universally appealing as warm therapy, many individuals find that alternating between heat and cold can maximize relief, allowing for a more comprehensive approach to symptom management.

The key to effectively using warm and cold therapy lies in understanding individual responses to each treatment. Some people may find that warm therapy works better for them, while others may prefer the invigorating effects of cold therapy. Experimenting with both methods can help individuals determine the best combination for their unique symptoms. It is advisable to apply heat or cold for 15 to 20 minutes at a time, allowing the body to respond to each treatment adequately. Keeping a journal of responses can also provide insights into which therapy is more effective at different times or under varying circumstances.

Incorporating warm and cold therapy into a broader self-care routine can enhance the overall management of Restless Legs Syndrome. These therapies can be easily integrated with other strategies, such as stretching exercises, mindfulness techniques, and lifestyle adjustments.

By adopting a holistic approach that includes a variety of treatment options, individuals can find a personalized strategy that significantly reduces the impact of RLS, allowing for a more comfortable and restful life.

How To Ease Restless Legs Syndrome

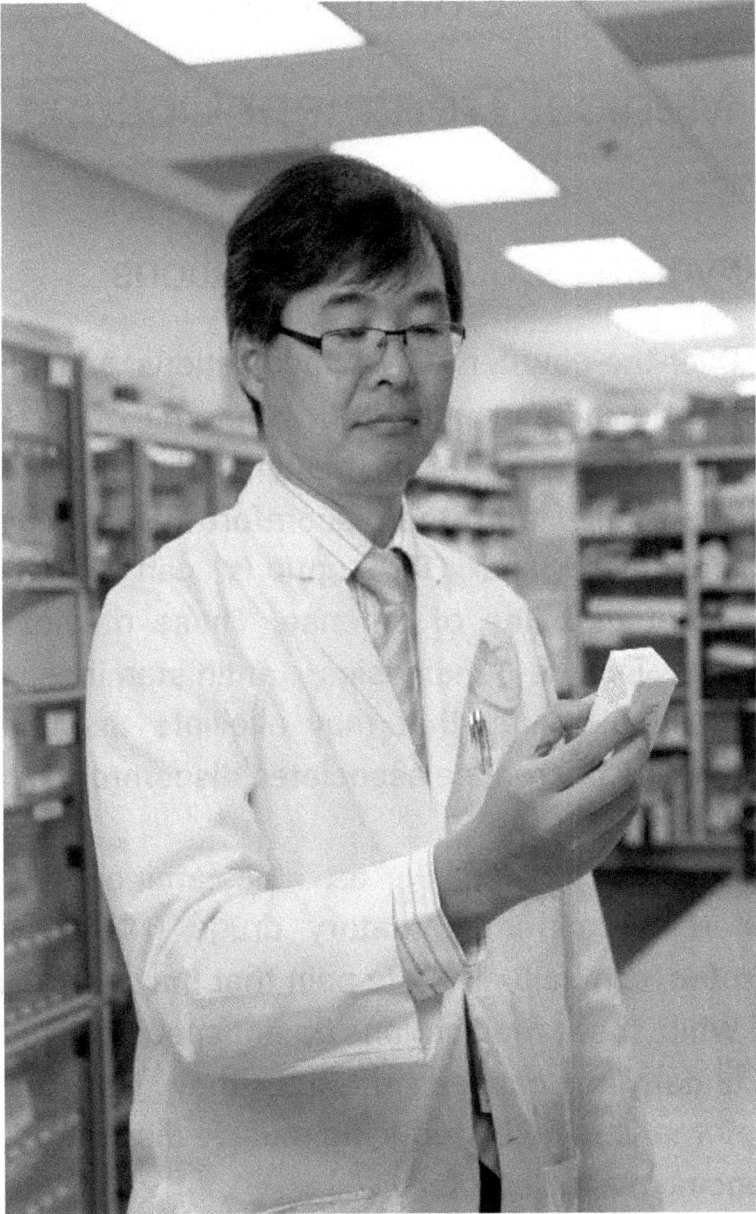

Effective Strategies for Relief

Chapter 5

Medical Treatment Options

Over-the-Counter Medications

Over-the-counter (OTC) medications can play a critical role in managing the symptoms of Restless Legs Syndrome (RLS). Many individuals seek immediate relief from the discomfort associated with this condition, and OTC options can provide a convenient first line of defense. These medications primarily include analgesics, antihistamines, and certain supplements that may alleviate the urge to move the legs or reduce associated discomfort.

Analgesics, such as acetaminophen or nonsteroidal anti-inflammatory drugs (NSAIDs) like ibuprofen, can help alleviate pain that may accompany RLS. While these medications do not specifically target the underlying causes of RLS, they can provide symptomatic relief by reducing muscle discomfort and enhancing overall comfort.

It is important to use these medications as directed and to consult with a healthcare professional if symptoms persist, as long-term use can lead to other health issues.

Antihistamines, commonly used to treat allergies, can also be beneficial for some individuals with RLS. Medications such as diphenhydramine, found in many OTC sleep aids, may help induce drowsiness and alleviate the uncomfortable sensations in the legs. However, caution is advised as these medications can cause sedation and may lead to dependency if used frequently. As with any medication, it is essential to monitor its effects and consult a healthcare provider if there are concerns about usage or side effects.

Certain dietary supplements, such as magnesium and iron, are also available over the counter and may assist in managing RLS symptoms. Magnesium plays a crucial role in muscle function and may help prevent muscle cramps, while iron is essential for proper nerve function. Individuals with RLS often have low levels of iron, so supplementation might help alleviate symptoms. It is advisable to undergo testing to determine iron levels before starting supplementation, as excessive iron intake can have adverse effects.

While OTC medications can provide temporary relief for RLS symptoms, they are not a cure. It is vital for individuals to adopt a comprehensive approach that includes lifestyle modifications, such as regular exercise, maintaining a consistent sleep schedule, and avoiding caffeine and nicotine. By combining these strategies with the appropriate use of OTC medications, individuals with RLS can significantly improve their quality of life and manage their symptoms more effectively.

Prescription Medications

Prescription medications play a crucial role in managing Restless Legs Syndrome (RLS) for many individuals. These medications are designed to alleviate the uncomfortable sensations and the overwhelming urge to move the legs, which can significantly disrupt daily life. When considering prescription options, it is essential to consult with a healthcare professional who can accurately diagnose RLS and recommend the most appropriate treatment based on individual symptoms and medical history.

Dopamine agonists are among the most commonly prescribed medications for RLS. These drugs work by stimulating dopamine receptors in the brain, which can help to reduce the severity of symptoms. Medications such as pramipexole and ropinirole are often effective in providing relief for patients. It is important to note that while these medications can be beneficial, they may also have side effects, including nausea, dizziness, and, in some cases, augmentation—where symptoms worsen over time. Monitoring and regular follow-ups with a healthcare provider are essential to adjusting dosages and ensuring the best outcomes.

Another class of medications used to treat RLS includes anticonvulsants, such as gabapentin and pregabalin. These medications can help to relieve the sensory disturbances associated with RLS by altering the way nerves send messages to the brain. This can lead to a reduction in the urge to move the legs and an improvement in overall comfort. As with dopamine agonists, it is crucial for patients to discuss potential side effects, such as drowsiness and weight gain, with their healthcare provider to weigh the benefits against any risks.

Iron supplements may also be prescribed for individuals with RLS who have low ferritin levels, as iron deficiency has been linked to the condition. In such cases, a healthcare provider may recommend iron therapy to address the deficiency, which can lead to an improvement in symptoms. Regular blood tests are often necessary to monitor iron levels and ensure safety during supplementation. It is essential to approach iron supplementation cautiously, as excessive iron can lead to other health complications.

Lastly, it is important to remember that prescription medications are often most effective when combined with lifestyle changes and non-pharmacological approaches. Patients should consider incorporating regular exercise, maintaining proper sleep hygiene, and avoiding certain stimulants like caffeine and nicotine. By taking a comprehensive approach to managing RLS, individuals can significantly improve their quality of life and find lasting relief from the symptoms that plague them. Always consult with a healthcare professional to create a tailored plan that addresses both medication and lifestyle modifications for optimal results.

Alternative Therapies

Alternative therapies for Restless Legs Syndrome (RLS) offer various approaches to alleviate symptoms and improve overall well-being. Many individuals seeking relief from RLS may find that conventional treatments do not fully address their needs or may come with undesirable side effects. As a result, exploring alternative therapies can provide additional options that complement standard medical care. These therapies often focus on holistic and integrative practices, emphasizing the connection between the mind and body.

One popular alternative therapy is acupuncture, a traditional Chinese medicine practice that involves inserting thin needles into specific points on the body. Studies have indicated that acupuncture may help reduce the severity of RLS symptoms by promoting relaxation and improving blood circulation. Some patients report a decrease in the urge to move their legs and an enhancement in sleep quality following acupuncture sessions. While individual results may vary, many find this non-invasive treatment a valuable addition to their RLS management plan.

Another approach gaining traction is the incorporation of dietary changes and nutritional supplements. Certain vitamins and minerals, such as iron, magnesium, and folate, play a crucial role in nerve function and muscle health. Individuals with RLS often experience deficiencies in these nutrients, which can exacerbate symptoms.

By focusing on a balanced diet rich in these essential nutrients or considering supplements, individuals may find significant relief. Additionally, herbal remedies like valerian root or passionflower have been used traditionally to promote relaxation and improve sleep quality, potentially benefiting those with RLS.

Mind-body practices, including yoga and meditation, have also shown promise in managing RLS symptoms. Yoga promotes flexibility, muscle relaxation, and stress reduction, which can alleviate the tension that often accompanies RLS. Practicing mindfulness meditation can help individuals manage anxiety and improve their overall sense of well-being, potentially reducing the frequency and intensity of RLS episodes.

Regular engagement in these practices fosters a greater awareness of bodily sensations and cultivates a sense of calm, which can be especially beneficial for those struggling with the discomfort of RLS.

Lastly, lifestyle modifications such as regular exercise, maintaining a consistent sleep schedule, and minimizing caffeine and alcohol consumption can play a significant role in managing RLS. Engaging in moderate physical activity can help improve circulation and reduce the severity of symptoms. Meanwhile, establishing a bedtime routine that promotes relaxation can enhance sleep quality, which is often disrupted by RLS. By integrating these alternative therapies and lifestyle changes into their daily routines, individuals may discover effective strategies for easing their RLS symptoms and improving their quality of life.

How To Ease Restless Legs Syndrome

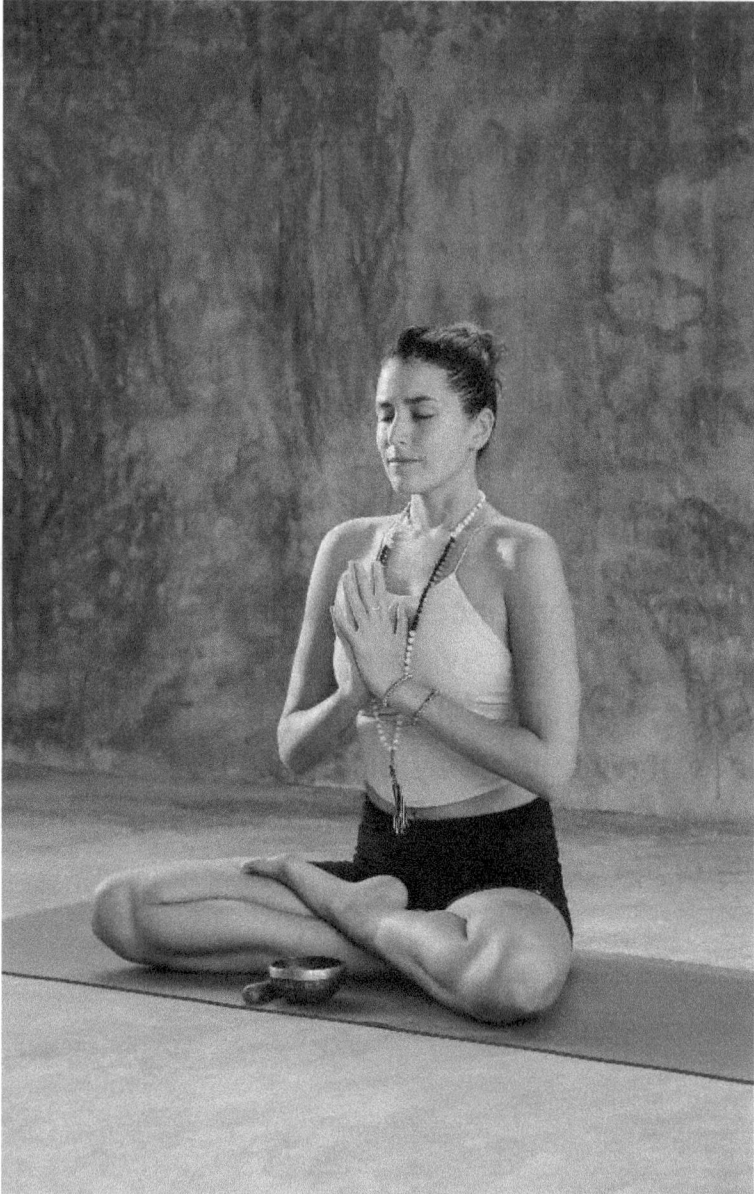

Chapter 6
Coping Strategies

Stress Management Techniques

Stress management plays a crucial role in alleviating the symptoms of Restless Legs Syndrome (RLS). Stress can exacerbate the discomfort associated with RLS, making effective stress management techniques essential for those seeking relief. Understanding how stress impacts the body and finding ways to mitigate it can lead to a significant reduction in RLS symptoms. This subchapter will explore various stress management techniques that can be beneficial for individuals dealing with RLS.

One effective technique for managing stress is mindfulness meditation. This practice encourages individuals to focus on the present moment, helping to reduce anxiety and promote relaxation. By incorporating mindfulness meditation into a daily routine, individuals with RLS can learn to calm their minds and bodies, which may contribute to a decrease in leg discomfort.

Simple breathing exercises, such as deep belly breathing, can also be integrated into mindfulness practices, providing immediate relief from stress and tension.

Physical activity is another powerful stress management technique. Engaging in regular exercise can significantly enhance mood and decrease stress levels. For individuals with RLS, low-impact activities such as walking, swimming, or yoga can be particularly beneficial.

These exercises not only help to relieve stress but also promote better circulation and muscle relaxation, which may alleviate some of the symptoms associated with RLS. Establishing a consistent exercise routine can serve as a proactive approach to managing both stress and RLS symptoms.

Another essential technique is establishing a consistent sleep schedule. Quality sleep is vital for overall well-being, and disruptions caused by RLS can lead to increased stress and anxiety. By creating a calming bedtime routine and adhering to a regular sleep schedule, individuals can improve their sleep quality.

Techniques such as limiting screen time before bed, creating a comfortable sleep environment, and practicing relaxation techniques can help prepare the body for restful sleep, ultimately reducing stress and the severity of RLS symptoms.

Finally, seeking social support can be an invaluable resource for stress management. Connecting with friends, family, or support groups can provide emotional relief and practical advice for managing RLS.

Sharing experiences and coping strategies with others who understand the condition can create a sense of community and reduce feelings of isolation. Whether through in-person gatherings or online forums, fostering these connections can be a vital part of a holistic approach to managing stress and easing the symptoms of RLS.

Mindfulness and Relaxation

Mindfulness and relaxation techniques can play a significant role in managing the discomfort associated with Restless Legs Syndrome (RLS).

These practices focus on reducing stress and promoting a sense of calm, which can be particularly beneficial for individuals experiencing the involuntary sensations often associated with RLS.

By incorporating mindfulness and relaxation into daily routines, individuals may find relief from symptoms and improve their overall quality of life.

Mindfulness involves being fully present in the moment and observing thoughts and sensations without judgment. This practice can help individuals with RLS to acknowledge their symptoms without becoming overwhelmed by them. Engaging in mindfulness meditation can provide a sense of control over the body's responses.

Techniques such as deep breathing, progressive muscle relaxation, and guided imagery can enhance this awareness, allowing individuals to shift their focus away from discomfort and toward relaxation.

Incorporating relaxation exercises into the daily routine can also alleviate RLS symptoms. Activities such as yoga and tai chi encourage gentle movement and stretching, which can help to reduce muscle tension and promote circulation.

These practices not only facilitate physical relaxation but also encourage mental tranquility, which is essential for managing stress levels that can exacerbate RLS symptoms. Regular practice of these exercises can lead to a greater sense of balance in both body and mind.

Establishing a nighttime routine that includes mindfulness and relaxation techniques can be particularly beneficial for those who experience increased RLS symptoms in the evening.

Creating a calming environment, free from distractions, can enhance the effectiveness of these practices. Techniques such as reading, taking a warm bath, or practicing gentle stretches can prepare the body for sleep and reduce the likelihood of RLS disturbances during the night.

In summary, integrating mindfulness and relaxation techniques into a comprehensive approach to managing Restless Legs Syndrome can offer significant benefits. By fostering an environment of calm and awareness, individuals may find it easier to cope with the challenges of RLS. As they develop these skills, they may not only experience relief from symptoms but also enjoy an enhanced sense of well-being and improved sleep quality.

Support Groups and Resources

Support groups and resources play a crucial role in managing Restless Legs Syndrome (RLS) by providing individuals with a sense of community and access to valuable information. These groups allow those affected by RLS to share their experiences, coping strategies, and emotional support. Connecting with others who understand the challenges of living with RLS can alleviate feelings of isolation and anxiety, making it easier to navigate the ups and downs of the condition. In addition to emotional support, these groups often provide practical tips and strategies that have worked for others, fostering a collaborative environment for finding relief.

There are various types of support groups available for individuals dealing with RLS. Online forums and social media groups are particularly beneficial for those who may have difficulty attending in-person meetings. These platforms allow for real-time sharing of experiences and solutions, making it easier to connect with a broader community. Additionally, many organizations focused on sleep disorders offer resources specifically tailored for RLS, including virtual meetings and webinars. These gatherings often feature experts in the field who can provide insights into the latest research and treatment options, helping members stay informed and empowered in their journey toward relief.

Local support groups can also be an invaluable resource for those seeking face-to-face interactions. Many hospitals, clinics, and community centers host regular meetings for individuals with RLS, allowing participants to build relationships and share their stories in a safe environment. These gatherings can foster a sense of belonging and encourage individuals to actively participate in their own care. Members often exchange information about local healthcare providers, treatments, and lifestyle changes that have proven effective in managing their symptoms.

In addition to peer-led support groups, various organizations offer educational resources that can aid in understanding and managing RLS. Websites dedicated to sleep disorders, such as the National Sleep Foundation and the RLS Foundation, provide a wealth of information, including articles, research studies, and treatment guidelines.

These resources can help individuals better understand their condition, recognize triggers, and implement practical strategies for symptom relief. Many organizations also provide access to newsletters, podcasts, and webinars, keeping members informed about new developments in RLS research and treatment options.

Lastly, it is essential to acknowledge the role of healthcare professionals in supporting individuals with RLS. Engaging with specialists, such as neurologists or sleep medicine experts, can provide valuable insights and personalized treatment plans. Healthcare providers can also recommend appropriate support groups or resources tailored to an individual's specific needs.

Building a supportive network that includes both peers and professionals can lead to a more comprehensive approach to managing RLS, ultimately improving the quality of life for those affected by this challenging condition.

How To Ease Restless Legs Syndrome

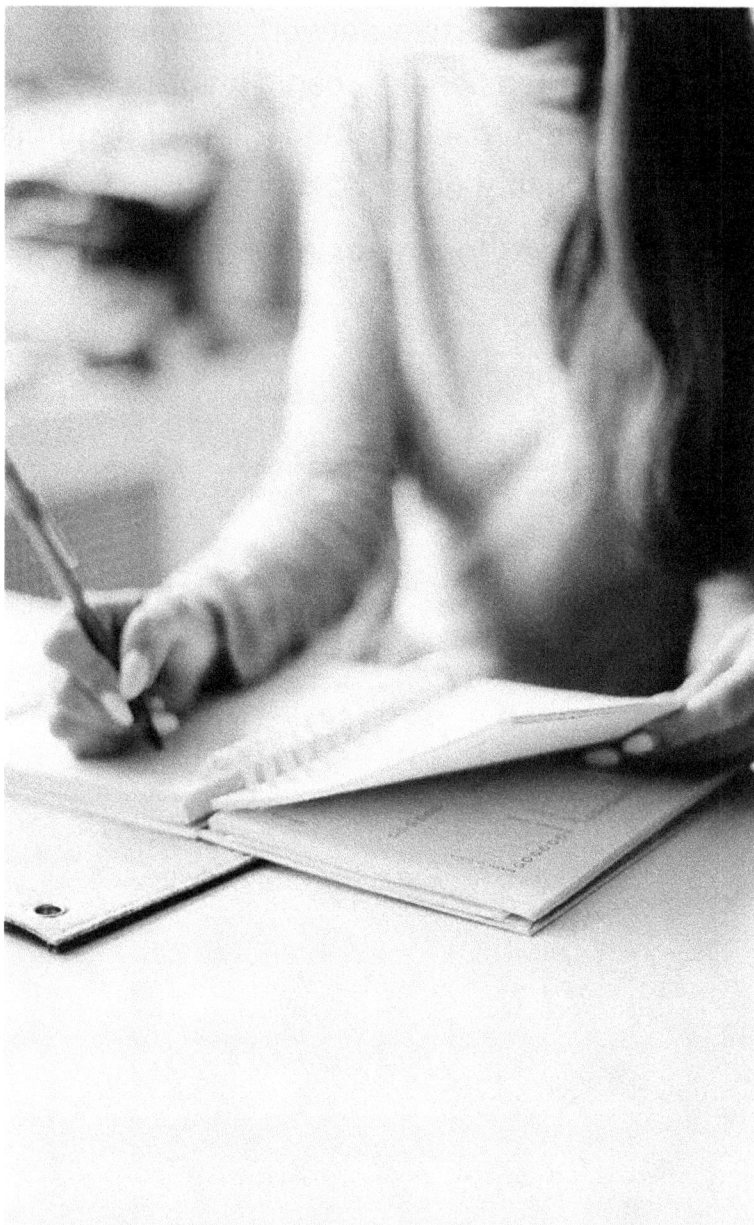

Effective Strategies for Relief

Chapter 7

Long-Term Management of Restless Legs Syndrome

Monitoring Symptoms

Monitoring symptoms is a crucial aspect of managing Restless Legs Syndrome (RLS). Individuals experiencing RLS often describe their symptoms as uncomfortable sensations in the legs, accompanied by an overwhelming urge to move. These sensations can vary in intensity and frequency, making it essential for patients to keep a detailed record of their experiences.

By documenting when and where symptoms occur, as well as their severity, individuals can identify patterns and triggers that exacerbate their condition. This information is invaluable when discussing treatment options with healthcare providers.

A symptom diary can be a useful tool in this process. Recording daily experiences allows individuals to track the frequency and severity of their symptoms over time. A diary should include details such as the time of day symptoms occur, how long they last, and any activities or lifestyle factors that may influence these sensations. This practice not only enhances self-awareness but also provides a tangible representation of the condition that can be shared with doctors. Healthcare professionals can better tailor treatment plans based on this comprehensive understanding of a patient's symptoms.

In addition to a symptom diary, individuals can benefit from using mobile apps designed for symptom tracking. Many of these apps allow users to log their symptoms conveniently and can even provide reminders for medication schedules. Some apps also offer features to track sleep quality and daily activities, which are important factors in RLS management. Analyzing this data can reveal correlations between lifestyle choices and symptom severity, empowering individuals to make informed decisions about their routines.

It is also essential to monitor the impact of lifestyle changes on RLS symptoms. Factors such as diet, exercise, and sleep hygiene can significantly influence symptom management. For example, individuals may notice that certain foods or beverages exacerbate their symptoms, while regular physical activity may help alleviate them. By being mindful of these connections, individuals can adopt healthier habits that may lead to a reduction in symptom severity.

Finally, regular check-ins with healthcare providers are vital for effective RLS management. Sharing symptom logs and observations can help clinicians assess the effectiveness of current treatments and make necessary adjustments.

This collaborative approach ensures that individuals receive personalized care tailored to their specific needs. Continuous monitoring of symptoms not only helps in managing RLS but also fosters a proactive mindset, empowering individuals to take charge of their health and well-being.

Adjusting Lifestyle as Needed

Adjusting lifestyle as needed is an essential component in managing Restless Legs Syndrome (RLS) effectively. Individuals experiencing RLS often find that certain lifestyle habits can exacerbate their symptoms, while others may provide relief. By making informed adjustments to daily routines, individuals can significantly reduce the frequency and intensity of their symptoms. This subchapter explores various lifestyle changes that can help ease the discomfort associated with RLS.

One of the most impactful lifestyle changes involves evaluating and improving sleep hygiene. Poor sleep quality can worsen RLS symptoms, creating a vicious cycle of discomfort and fatigue. Establishing a regular sleep schedule, creating a relaxing bedtime routine, and ensuring a comfortable sleep environment can contribute to better rest. It is also beneficial to limit screen time before bed and avoid stimulants such as caffeine and nicotine in the hours leading up to sleep. By prioritizing sleep health, individuals can often find themselves managing RLS symptoms more effectively.

Nutrition plays a vital role in overall well-being and can influence RLS symptoms as well. A balanced diet rich in iron, magnesium, and folate is particularly beneficial, as deficiencies in these nutrients have been linked to RLS. Incorporating foods such as leafy greens, nuts, seeds, and lean proteins can help support nerve function and reduce the severity of symptoms. Additionally, staying hydrated and minimizing processed foods can contribute to improved health outcomes. Paying attention to dietary choices can be a simple yet powerful strategy in managing RLS.

Regular physical activity is another crucial aspect of lifestyle adjustment for those coping with RLS. Engaging in moderate exercise can enhance circulation and promote relaxation, which may alleviate symptoms. Activities such as walking, cycling, or yoga can be particularly beneficial, as they not only improve physical fitness but also reduce stress levels. However, it is essential to find a balance, as excessive or high-intensity exercise close to bedtime can sometimes worsen symptoms. Establishing a consistent exercise routine can empower individuals to take control of their RLS.

Lastly, managing stress through mindfulness and relaxation techniques can offer significant relief from RLS symptoms. Stress is known to exacerbate various health conditions, including RLS. Techniques such as deep breathing, meditation, and progressive muscle relaxation can help reduce anxiety and promote a sense of calm. Creating a supportive environment, whether through social connections or engaging in hobbies, can further enhance emotional well-being. By addressing stressors and incorporating relaxation practices into daily life, individuals can create a more conducive atmosphere for managing RLS effectively.

Working with Healthcare Providers

When dealing with Restless Legs Syndrome (RLS), collaboration with healthcare providers is a crucial step in managing symptoms effectively. Engaging with professionals such as primary care physicians, neurologists, and sleep specialists can provide individuals with a comprehensive approach to treatment. These experts can evaluate symptoms, rule out potential underlying conditions, and recommend appropriate interventions tailored to each person's unique needs.

Building a strong relationship with healthcare providers fosters open communication, allowing individuals to express their concerns and preferences regarding treatment options.

Before visiting a healthcare provider, it is helpful for individuals to prepare by keeping a detailed symptom diary. This diary should document the frequency, duration, and severity of RLS symptoms, as well as any factors that may exacerbate or alleviate them. Noting lifestyle habits, such as sleep patterns, dietary choices, and physical activity levels, can also provide valuable insights. This information not only aids healthcare providers in making an accurate diagnosis but also helps in formulating an effective treatment plan. Being forthcoming about any other medical conditions or medications being taken is essential, as these can influence treatment decisions.

Healthcare providers often recommend a variety of treatment options based on the severity of RLS symptoms. Lifestyle modifications are typically the first line of defense, including regular exercise, maintaining a consistent sleep schedule, and avoiding caffeine and alcohol. For some individuals, these changes alone may significantly alleviate symptoms.

However, for others, more intensive treatments may be necessary. Healthcare providers can prescribe medications specifically approved for RLS or suggest off-label use of certain drugs that have shown efficacy in managing symptoms. Understanding the potential benefits and risks of these medications is vital for informed decision-making.

In addition to medication and lifestyle changes, healthcare providers may suggest complementary therapies. These can include physical therapy, acupuncture, or certain relaxation techniques aimed at reducing stress and promoting better sleep quality. Engaging in discussions about these alternative methods can lead to a more holistic approach to managing RLS. Patients should feel empowered to ask questions and explore various treatment modalities, as a collaborative effort can enhance the overall effectiveness of the management plan.

Regular follow-ups with healthcare providers are essential for monitoring the effectiveness of the chosen strategies and making necessary adjustments. As symptoms may evolve over time, maintaining an ongoing dialogue ensures that individuals receive the most appropriate and effective care.

It is important to communicate any changes in symptoms or side effects experienced from treatments. This proactive approach fosters a partnership with healthcare providers that can lead to improved outcomes and a better quality of life for those living with Restless Legs Syndrome.

How To Ease Restless Legs Syndrome

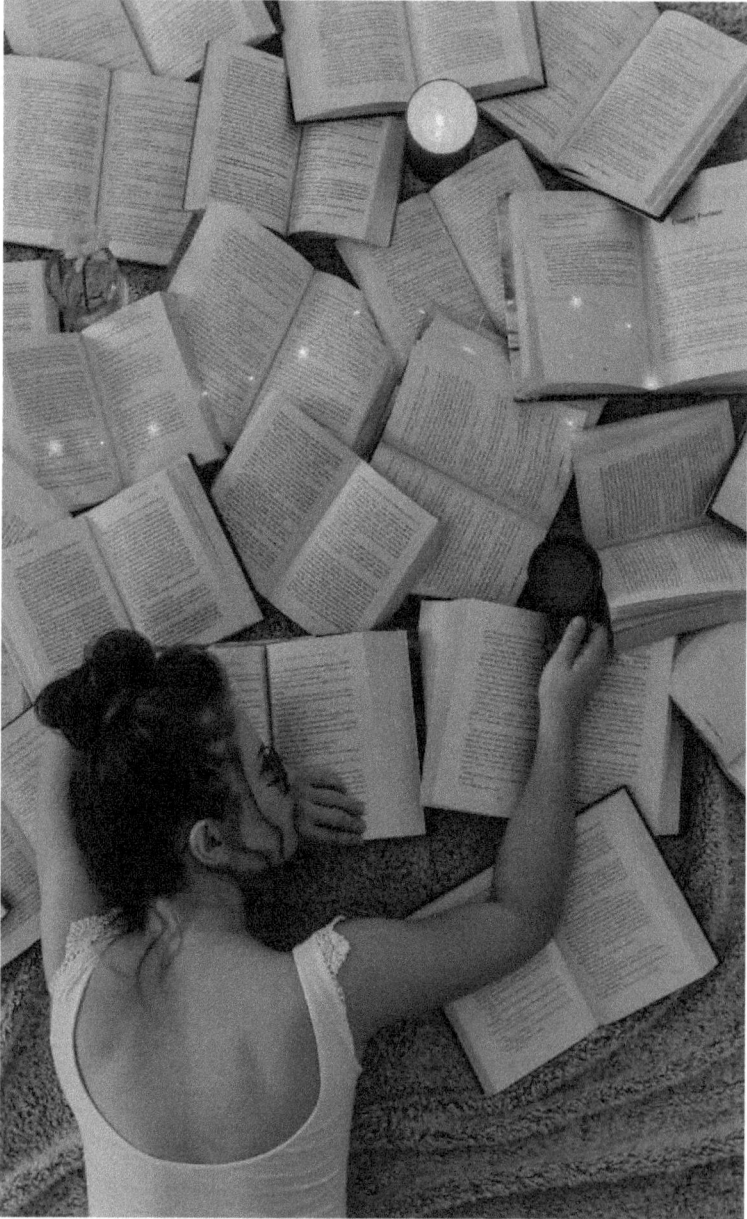

Chapter 8

Myths and Misconceptions

Common Myths About RLS

Restless Legs Syndrome (RLS) is often surrounded by misconceptions that can lead to misunderstanding and mismanagement of the condition. One common myth is that RLS only occurs in older adults. While it is true that the prevalence of RLS increases with age, it can affect individuals of all ages, including children and young adults. This misconception may prevent younger individuals experiencing symptoms from seeking help, causing unnecessary discomfort and a delay in obtaining effective treatment.

Another prevalent myth is that RLS is merely a psychological condition. Many people believe that the symptoms of RLS, which include uncomfortable sensations in the legs and an overwhelming urge to move them, are solely the result of anxiety or stress. In reality, RLS is a neurological disorder with a biological basis.

It is often associated with imbalances in dopamine, a neurotransmitter involved in controlling muscle movements. Understanding that RLS has a physiological component is crucial for those affected to seek appropriate medical advice and treatment options.

A third myth suggests that lifestyle changes have no impact on RLS symptoms. While it is true that some individuals may require medication for severe cases, many people can experience significant relief through lifestyle modifications.

Factors such as regular exercise, good sleep hygiene, and dietary adjustments can play a vital role in managing symptoms. Believing that RLS is unchangeable may lead individuals to overlook these effective strategies, ultimately affecting their quality of life.

Another misconception is that RLS is a rare condition. In fact, studies estimate that RLS affects approximately 5 to 10 percent of the population, making it relatively common.

This myth can lead to feelings of isolation for those who experience RLS, as they may believe they are alone in their struggles. Increased awareness and understanding of the condition can help individuals realize they are part of a larger community and encourage them to share their experiences and seek support.

Finally, some believe that RLS is only a nighttime issue. While the symptoms are often more pronounced during periods of rest, RLS can also affect individuals during the day, particularly when sitting for extended periods. This misconception can result in a lack of understanding of the daily challenges faced by those with RLS. Recognizing that the condition can disrupt both day and night allows for a more comprehensive approach to treatment and symptom management, leading to better outcomes for those affected.

Clarifying Misconceptions

Restless Legs Syndrome (RLS) is often misunderstood, leading to misconceptions that can hinder effective management of the condition. One common myth is that RLS is merely a psychological issue or a result of anxiety.

While stress can exacerbate symptoms, RLS is primarily a neurological disorder characterized by an uncontrollable urge to move the legs. This urge typically arises during periods of inactivity, particularly in the evening or at night, and is often accompanied by uncomfortable sensations.

Understanding the neurological basis of RLS is crucial for recognizing it as a legitimate medical condition deserving of attention and treatment.

Another prevalent misconception is that RLS only affects older adults. While it is true that the incidence of RLS increases with age, the syndrome can affect individuals of all ages, including children. Genetic factors play a significant role, as RLS often runs in families.

In fact, primary RLS, which has no identifiable cause, is frequently inherited. By acknowledging that younger individuals can also experience RLS, we can foster greater awareness and encourage those affected to seek appropriate help, regardless of their age.

How To Ease Restless Legs Syndrome

Many people believe that lifestyle changes have little impact on RLS symptoms. However, research indicates that certain modifications can significantly alleviate discomfort. Regular physical activity, a healthy diet, and good sleep hygiene can all contribute to reducing RLS symptoms. For instance, engaging in moderate exercise has been shown to improve circulation and decrease the severity of symptoms.

Additionally, avoiding caffeine, nicotine, and alcohol, especially in the evening, can help manage RLS more effectively. These lifestyle adjustments should be viewed as complementary strategies that enhance overall well-being and symptom relief.

Some individuals may assume that medication is the only solution for RLS. While pharmacological treatments can be effective, they are not the sole option available. There are various non-pharmacological approaches that can provide significant relief, such as massage, warm baths, and the use of heating pads or cold compresses. These methods can help soothe the legs and reduce the urge to move.

Furthermore, engaging in relaxation techniques like yoga or meditation can also be beneficial in managing symptoms. Exploring a combination of treatments can lead to a more personalized and effective management plan.

Finally, it is important to dispel the notion that RLS is a trivial condition that does not warrant medical attention. The impact of RLS on quality of life can be profound, affecting sleep, work, and overall emotional well-being.

Many individuals with RLS experience significant distress and fatigue due to disrupted sleep patterns. Recognizing the seriousness of RLS encourages those affected to seek help from healthcare professionals who can provide guidance on appropriate treatment options.

By clarifying these misconceptions, individuals can take empowered steps towards managing their RLS and improving their quality of life.

Evidence-Based Understanding

Restless Legs Syndrome (RLS) is a neurological disorder characterized by an uncontrollable urge to move the legs, often accompanied by uncomfortable sensations. The symptoms typically worsen during periods of inactivity and can significantly disrupt sleep. Understanding RLS from an evidence-based perspective is crucial for developing effective strategies for relief.

Research indicates that RLS may be linked to genetic factors, iron deficiency, and other underlying medical conditions. A comprehensive understanding of these factors can empower individuals to seek appropriate treatment and lifestyle changes.

Numerous studies have highlighted the role of iron levels in the development and severity of RLS symptoms. Iron is essential for dopamine production, a neurotransmitter that plays a critical role in controlling movement. Low iron levels in the brain can lead to increased RLS symptoms.

Research has shown that individuals with RLS often have lower serum ferritin levels, which is a marker of iron storage in the body. For those suffering from RLS, monitoring iron levels through blood tests and considering dietary adjustments or supplements may provide significant relief.

Genetic predisposition is another area of focus in the study of RLS. Meta-analyses have identified several gene variants that are associated with an increased risk of developing the condition. Understanding the hereditary nature of RLS can help individuals recognize their likelihood of experiencing symptoms and encourage them to take proactive measures. Moreover, family history can provide insights into the potential effectiveness of various treatments, as certain responses to medication may run in families.

Lifestyle factors also play a pivotal role in managing RLS symptoms. Evidence suggests that regular physical activity, proper sleep hygiene, and avoidance of stimulants such as caffeine and nicotine can mitigate the severity of RLS.

Engaging in moderate exercise can improve overall circulation and reduce discomfort in the legs. Furthermore, establishing a consistent sleep routine can help individuals achieve better rest, which is essential for managing RLS. Research supports the idea that a holistic approach, combining lifestyle changes with medical intervention, can yield the best outcomes for those affected by RLS.

Finally, emerging therapies and treatments continue to evolve based on ongoing research. Medications such as dopamine agonists and anticonvulsants have shown efficacy in alleviating symptoms for many patients.

Additionally, non-pharmacological interventions, including cognitive behavioral therapy and mindfulness practices, are gaining recognition for their potential benefits. As the scientific community continues to explore the complexities of RLS, individuals seeking relief can remain hopeful that evidence-based strategies will lead to effective management and improved quality of life.

How To Ease Restless Legs Syndrome

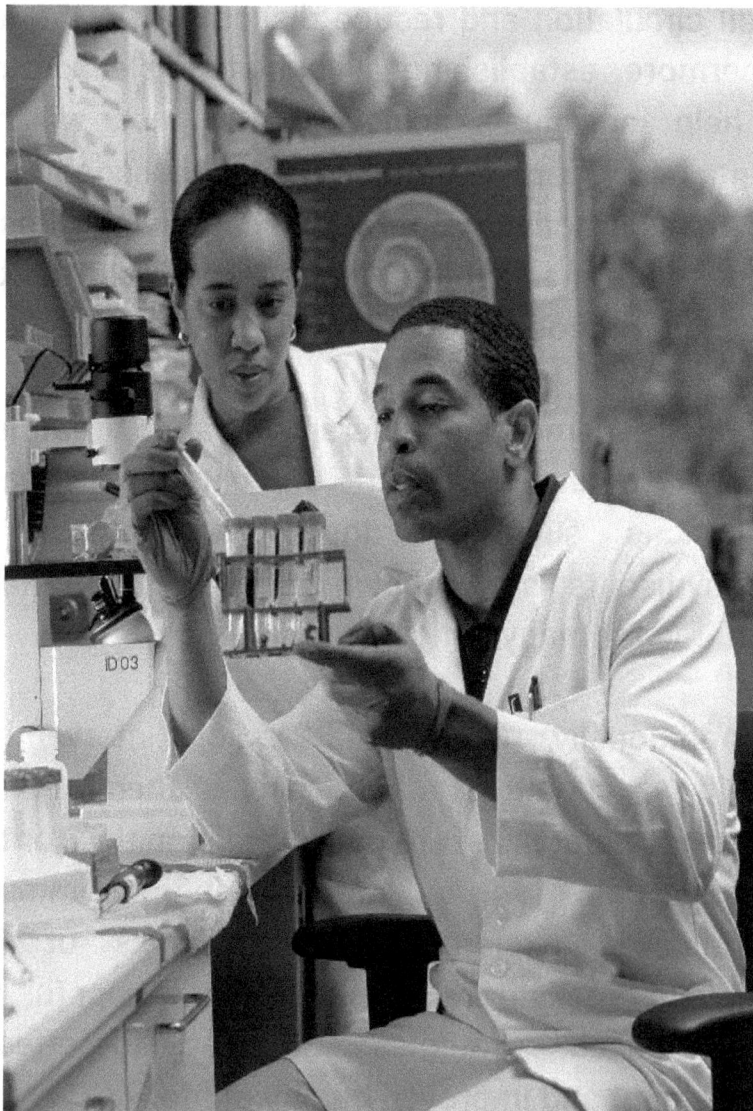

Effective Strategies for Relief

Chapter 9

Future Directions in RLS Research

Ongoing Studies

Ongoing studies on Restless Legs Syndrome (RLS) are crucial for enhancing our understanding of this condition and improving treatment options. Researchers worldwide are investigating various aspects of RLS, including its underlying mechanisms, genetic predispositions, and the effectiveness of different therapeutic approaches.

These studies aim to uncover the reasons behind the symptoms, which can vary significantly from person to person, thus paving the way for more personalized treatment plans.

One area of focus in current research is the role of iron deficiency in RLS. Several studies indicate that low iron levels in the brain may contribute to the development of symptoms. Researchers are exploring the effects of iron supplementation and its potential to alleviate RLS symptoms, particularly in individuals with documented iron deficiency. This line of inquiry is especially relevant as it offers a straightforward intervention that could lead to significant improvements for many patients.

Additionally, the impact of lifestyle modifications on RLS is being rigorously examined. Researchers are studying how factors such as diet, exercise, and sleep hygiene influence the severity and frequency of symptoms.

Preliminary findings suggest that certain dietary changes, regular physical activity, and improved sleep practices can lead to substantial relief for some individuals. As these studies progress, they could provide essential insights into non-pharmacological strategies that can complement existing treatments.

Pharmacological interventions continue to be a significant focus of ongoing studies as well. New medications are being tested for their efficacy and safety in treating RLS. This includes both traditional dopaminergic treatments and novel approaches that target different neurotransmitter systems. By evaluating the long-term effects of these medications, researchers hope to identify options that not only provide relief but also minimize side effects, enhancing the overall quality of life for those affected by the syndrome.

Finally, the exploration of genetic factors associated with RLS is a burgeoning field of research. Understanding the genetic basis of RLS could lead to the identification of at-risk populations and the development of targeted therapies.

As genomic studies advance, they may reveal specific genetic markers that correlate with the severity of symptoms or response to treatment. This knowledge could transform how RLS is approached, allowing for more tailored and effective management strategies for individuals suffering from this challenging condition.

Innovations in Treatment

Innovations in treatment for Restless Legs Syndrome (RLS) have advanced significantly in recent years, offering new hope for those affected by this often debilitating condition. Traditional therapies, including dopaminergic medications, have been the cornerstone of RLS management, but recent developments have expanded the arsenal of options available to patients. These innovations not only aim to alleviate symptoms but also address the underlying mechanisms of the disorder, leading to more effective and personalized treatment strategies.

One notable advancement is the emergence of non-dopaminergic medications. For patients who experience side effects from traditional treatments or have inadequate responses, drugs such as gabapentin and pregabalin have shown promise. These medications target different neurotransmitter pathways and can help reduce the sensory disturbances associated with RLS. Clinical studies have demonstrated their efficacy in improving sleep quality and reducing the urge to move, providing a valuable alternative for individuals seeking relief.

In addition to pharmacological innovations, lifestyle interventions have gained recognition as effective components of RLS management. Recent research emphasizes the role of diet, exercise, and sleep hygiene in mitigating symptoms. For instance, incorporating regular physical activity and a balanced diet rich in iron and magnesium may improve overall symptoms. Furthermore, cognitive-behavioral therapy (CBT) is being explored as a complementary approach, helping individuals to develop coping strategies and address anxiety often associated with RLS.

Technological advancements have also made strides in the treatment of RLS. Wearable devices and mobile applications that track symptoms and sleep patterns are increasingly being integrated into management plans. These tools allow patients to monitor their conditions more closely and provide valuable data for healthcare providers to tailor treatments effectively. Additionally, neuromodulation techniques, such as transcranial magnetic stimulation (TMS) and peripheral nerve stimulation, are being investigated for their potential to alter the neural pathways involved in RLS, offering new avenues of relief.

Finally, ongoing research continues to shed light on the genetic and environmental factors contributing to RLS. Understanding these elements paves the way for innovative treatments that target the root causes of the syndrome rather than just the symptoms. As the field progresses, it is anticipated that more personalized and effective treatment options will emerge, empowering individuals with RLS to take control of their symptoms and improve their quality of life. The future of RLS management looks promising, with a focus on a comprehensive approach that combines medical, lifestyle, and technological innovations.

What Lies Ahead for RLS Patients

As research into Restless Legs Syndrome (RLS) continues to evolve, patients can anticipate a future with improved understanding and treatment options. Ongoing studies have expanded knowledge about the underlying mechanisms of RLS, which may lead to targeted therapies that address the root causes rather than just alleviating symptoms.

This deeper understanding is crucial, as it allows for the development of personalized treatment plans that can significantly enhance the quality of life for those affected by RLS.

In the coming years, advancements in pharmacological treatments are likely to emerge. Current therapies focus on managing symptoms through medications such as dopaminergic agents, opioids, and anticonvulsants. However, researchers are exploring new drug classes and formulations that could offer more effective relief with fewer side effects. These innovations may also include longer-acting medications that reduce the frequency of doses patients must take, thereby simplifying their treatment regimens.

Moreover, lifestyle modifications and non-pharmacological approaches are gaining attention as integral components of RLS management. Techniques such as cognitive behavioral therapy, mindfulness practices, and regular exercise have shown promise in mitigating symptoms.

As awareness about these strategies increases, healthcare providers may begin to incorporate them more regularly into treatment plans, empowering patients to take an active role in managing their condition through holistic approaches.

Technological advancements also hold exciting potential for RLS patients. Wearable devices that monitor sleep patterns, movement, and symptoms could provide valuable data for both patients and healthcare professionals. This information can lead to more tailored treatment approaches, as well as allow patients to track their progress and identify triggers that worsen their symptoms. Mobile applications designed for symptom management and education could further support patients in their journey toward relief.

Finally, community support and advocacy efforts are expected to grow, fostering a more informed and supportive environment for those living with RLS. Organizations dedicated to raising awareness and funding research initiatives will play a critical role in shaping the future of RLS care.

By connecting patients with resources, educational materials, and support networks, a collective approach can enhance the overall experience of managing RLS, offering hope and relief to many who struggle with this challenging condition.

How To Ease Restless Legs Syndrome

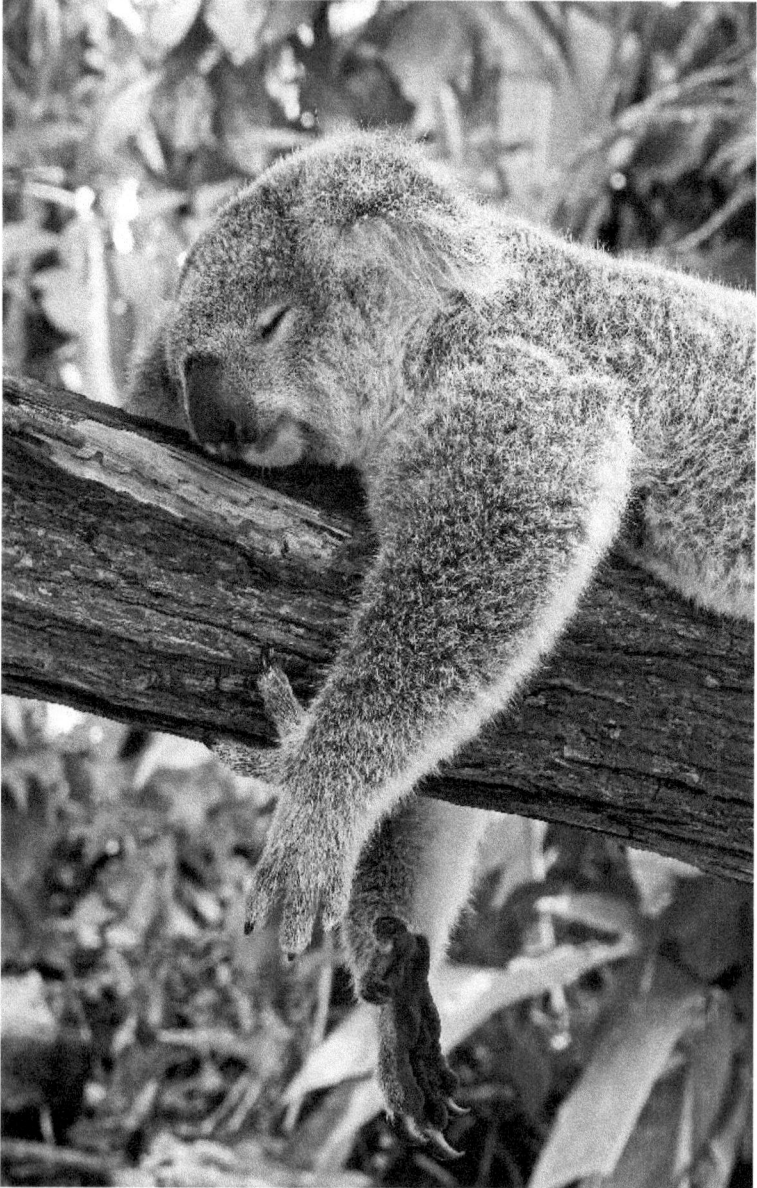

Chapter 10

Conclusion

Recap of Effective Strategies

Restless Legs Syndrome (RLS) can significantly impact the quality of life for those affected by it. To effectively manage the symptoms of RLS, various strategies have proven to be beneficial. These strategies encompass lifestyle modifications, dietary changes, and the use of certain therapies that can alleviate the discomfort associated with this condition.

By revisiting these effective approaches, individuals can better understand how to implement them in their daily routines for optimal relief.

One of the primary strategies for easing RLS symptoms is maintaining a consistent sleep schedule. Establishing a regular bedtime and wake-up time helps regulate the body's internal clock, which can reduce the severity of symptoms.

Creating a calming bedtime routine, such as engaging in relaxation techniques or gentle stretching, can also prepare the body for sleep. It is essential to ensure that the sleep environment is conducive to rest, minimizing disturbances that can exacerbate RLS.

Dietary considerations play a crucial role in managing RLS. Certain nutrients, such as iron, magnesium, and folate, are believed to influence the severity of symptoms. Incorporating foods rich in these nutrients, such as leafy greens, nuts, and whole grains, may provide relief.

Additionally, individuals should be mindful of their caffeine and alcohol intake, as both substances can trigger or worsen symptoms. Staying hydrated and maintaining a balanced diet can further support overall well-being and help mitigate RLS effects.

Physical activity is another vital component in managing RLS. Regular exercise not only promotes better circulation but also helps to reduce stress and anxiety, which can trigger symptoms. Activities such as walking, swimming, and yoga are particularly beneficial for individuals with RLS.

It is important to engage in these activities during the day, as exercising too close to bedtime can lead to difficulty falling asleep. Finding an enjoyable form of exercise can make it easier to maintain a consistent routine.

In some cases, medical interventions may be necessary to manage RLS effectively. Consulting with a healthcare provider can lead to personalized treatment options, which may include medications or supplements aimed at alleviating symptoms. Additionally, exploring alternative therapies, such as acupuncture or massage, may offer additional relief.

By combining these medical approaches with lifestyle and dietary changes, individuals can create a comprehensive management plan tailored to their specific needs. Reassessing these effective strategies regularly can help individuals adapt and refine their methods for optimal relief from Restless Legs Syndrome.

Encouragement for Those Affected

Living with Restless Legs Syndrome (RLS) can be a challenging experience, but it is essential to remember that you are not alone. Many individuals face similar struggles, and understanding that this condition affects countless others can provide solace. The shared experiences of those with RLS can foster a sense of community and belonging. Connecting with support groups, both online and in-person, may help alleviate feelings of isolation and provide a platform for exchanging tips and coping strategies.

One of the most effective ways to combat the challenges of RLS is to educate yourself about the condition. Knowledge is empowering, and understanding the underlying mechanisms of RLS can provide clarity and direction. Researching potential triggers, symptoms, and effective management strategies can help you take control of your situation. Awareness of how factors like diet, sleep hygiene, and physical activity influence RLS can guide you in making informed lifestyle choices that may mitigate symptoms.

In addition to education, exploring holistic approaches can be beneficial. Many individuals have found relief through relaxation techniques, such as yoga, meditation, or deep-breathing exercises. Incorporating these practices into your daily routine can not only help reduce RLS symptoms but also improve overall well-being. Finding activities that help you unwind and reduce stress is crucial, as heightened anxiety can exacerbate the symptoms of RLS.

Support from family and friends plays a vital role in managing RLS. Open communication about your condition can foster understanding and encourage loved ones to be more supportive as you navigate your journey. Whether it's simple gestures like offering a foot massage or creating a calming environment for relaxation, having a supportive network can make a significant difference in managing stress and enhancing your quality of life.

Finally, remember that progress may take time, and it is essential to be patient with yourself. Celebrate small victories along the way, whether it's a night of restful sleep or successfully implementing a new strategy.

Each step you take towards understanding and managing RLS is a step towards a more comfortable and fulfilling life. Embrace the journey, and know that with persistence and the right resources, relief is possible.

Final Thoughts on Living with RLS

Living with Restless Legs Syndrome (RLS) can be a challenging experience, affecting not only physical comfort but also emotional well-being. Individuals often find themselves grappling with the persistent urge to move their legs, particularly during periods of inactivity or at night. This can lead to disturbed sleep patterns, fatigue, and a decrease in overall quality of life. Understanding the complexities of RLS is crucial for those seeking effective strategies for relief, as it allows for better management of symptoms and a more fulfilling lifestyle.

One of the most effective approaches to managing RLS involves establishing a consistent daily routine. This includes maintaining regular sleep patterns, engaging in moderate exercise, and adopting relaxation techniques.

How To Ease Restless Legs Syndrome

Sleep hygiene practices, such as creating a comfortable sleep environment and limiting screen time before bed, can significantly improve sleep quality. Additionally, incorporating gentle stretching or yoga into a daily routine can help alleviate symptoms. By making these changes, individuals can create a more stable foundation for managing RLS.

Dietary choices also play a vital role in managing Restless Legs Syndrome. Nutritional deficiencies, particularly in iron, magnesium, and folate, can exacerbate symptoms. Therefore, it is essential to focus on a balanced diet rich in these nutrients. Foods such as leafy greens, nuts, seeds, and lean proteins can contribute to improved overall health and potentially reduce RLS symptoms. Staying hydrated and minimizing caffeine and alcohol intake can further enhance the effectiveness of dietary strategies in managing symptoms.

In addition to lifestyle and dietary modifications, seeking medical advice is crucial for those experiencing moderate to severe symptoms. Healthcare professionals can provide valuable insights and potential treatment options, including medications specifically designed to alleviate RLS symptoms.

It is vital for individuals to communicate openly with their healthcare providers about their experiences, as this can lead to a more tailored treatment approach. Exploring various treatment modalities can empower individuals to find the most effective strategies for their unique situations.

Ultimately, living with Restless Legs Syndrome requires a multifaceted approach. By combining lifestyle changes, dietary adjustments, and professional guidance, individuals can take proactive steps toward managing their symptoms. It is essential to remain patient and persistent, as finding the right combination of strategies may take time. With the right tools and support, individuals can navigate the challenges of RLS and work toward a more comfortable and fulfilling life.

Author Notes & Acknowledgments

First and foremost, I would like to express my deepest gratitude to the people who inspired and supported me throughout the journey of writing this book. This project would not have been possible without their unwavering belief in me and their invaluable contributions.

To my wife, thank you for your constant encouragement and understanding. Your love and support have been my anchor during the challenging times of researching and writing this book. Your belief in my ability to make a difference in people's lives has been my driving force.

I would also like to disclose that this book contains some renewed artificial intelligence-generated content. I really appreciate very recent technological innovation by outstanding scientists and of course our reader's understanding.

Lastly, I want to express my deepest gratitude to the readers of this book. I sincerely hope the strategies and methods outlined within these pages will provide you with the knowledge and tools needed to truly make your life much better. Your commitment to seeking any good solutions and willingness to explore multiple methods is commendable.

Author Bio

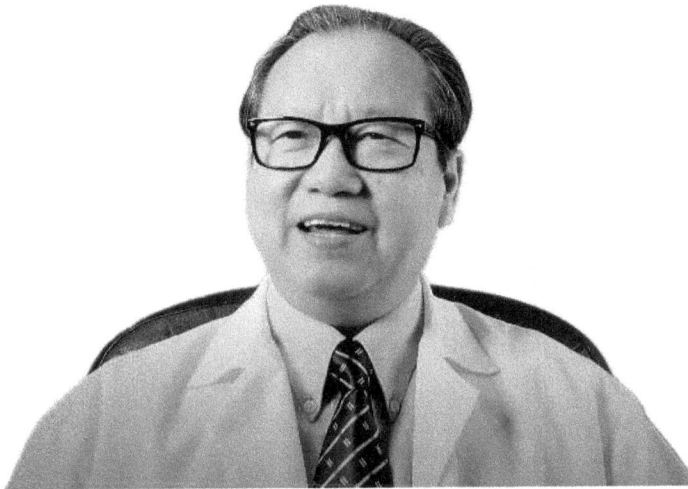

Johnson Wu earned his MD in 1982. With over 40 years of clinical experience, he has worked in hospitals in Zhejiang and Shanghai, China, as well as the Royal Marsden Hospital (part of Imperial College) in London, UK. Upon the recommendation of Sir Aaron Klug, the president of The Royal Society and a Nobel Prize winner in Chemistry, Dr. Wu was honorably awarded a British Royal Society Fellowship. He has published over 100 medical books in many countries and currently practices medicine in Canada.

www.ingramcontent.com/pod-product-compliance
Lightning Source LLC
Chambersburg PA
CBHW060252030426
42335CB00014B/1663

www.ingramcontent.com/pod-product-compliance
Lightning Source LLC
Chambersburg PA
CBHW060252030426
42335CB00014B/1663